Mariana Marquezan
Amanda Carneiro da Cunha
Lincoln Issamu Nojima

Miniscrew covering to prevent traumatic lesions

AF153318

Mariana Marquezan
Amanda Carneiro da Cunha
Lincoln Issamu Nojima

Miniscrew covering to prevent traumatic lesions

LAP LAMBERT Academic Publishing

Impressum / Imprint
Bibliografische Information der Deutschen Nationalbibliothek: Die Deutsche Nationalbibliothek verzeichnet diese Publikation in der Deutschen Nationalbibliografie; detaillierte bibliografische Daten sind im Internet über http://dnb.d-nb.de abrufbar.
Alle in diesem Buch genannten Marken und Produktnamen unterliegen warenzeichen-, marken- oder patentrechtlichem Schutz bzw. sind Warenzeichen oder eingetragene Warenzeichen der jeweiligen Inhaber. Die Wiedergabe von Marken, Produktnamen, Gebrauchsnamen, Handelsnamen, Warenbezeichnungen u.s.w. in diesem Werk berechtigt auch ohne besondere Kennzeichnung nicht zu der Annahme, dass solche Namen im Sinne der Warenzeichen- und Markenschutzgesetzgebung als frei zu betrachten wären und daher von jedermann benutzt werden dürften.

Bibliographic information published by the Deutsche Nationalbibliothek: The Deutsche Nationalbibliothek lists this publication in the Deutsche Nationalbibliografie; detailed bibliographic data are available in the Internet at http://dnb.d-nb.de.
Any brand names and product names mentioned in this book are subject to trademark, brand or patent protection and are trademarks or registered trademarks of their respective holders. The use of brand names, product names, common names, trade names, product descriptions etc. even without a particular marking in this work is in no way to be construed to mean that such names may be regarded as unrestricted in respect of trademark and brand protection legislation and could thus be used by anyone.

Coverbild / Cover image: www.ingimage.com

Verlag / Publisher:
LAP LAMBERT Academic Publishing
ist ein Imprint der / is a trademark of
OmniScriptum GmbH & Co. KG
Heinrich-Böcking-Str. 6-8, 66121 Saarbrücken, Deutschland / Germany
Email: info@lap-publishing.com

Herstellung: siehe letzte Seite /
Printed at: see last page
ISBN: 978-3-659-37227-8

Dedicated to the Professors of the Orthodontics Department of the Federal University of Rio de Janeiro (UFRJ) in appreciation of the teachings passed on to us, and their contribution to Brazilian Orthodontics.

Acknowledgments

The authors would like to thank Dr. Maria Teresa Villela Romanos for her assistance with the cytotoxicity experiments and Dr. Amanda Osório Ayres de Freitas, who co-authored the manuscript that originated this book.

TABLE OF CONTENTS

1.   The use of miniscrews in Orthodontics and the importance of covering them

Since the creation of the specialty of Orthodontics, proper anchorage control has been recognized as an important factor for achieving excellent results in treatment[1]. Anchorage materializes the physical concept of action and reaction: if the anchorage unit used does not offer adequate resistance, undesirable tooth movement will occur[1]. Orthodontic anchorage is usually achieved by a tooth or group of teeth that supports the movement of other elements[2]. Traditionally, this can be enhanced by increasing the number of teeth, using auxiliary intra-oral appliances and/or extra-oral devices[3]. However, some cases such as severe asymmetries, multiple dental losses or extensive periodontal involvement, can benefit from the use of skeletal anchorage[2], because this allows the achievement of tooth movement in three dimensions with minimal effects on other teeth[3]. Adults or non-compliant patients are also benefited from this system.

In 1907, Angle proposed that a static base would represent the ideal anchorage[1]. But it was only as from the 1980s that different devices have been used for skeletal anchorage in humans: vitallium screws[4], dental implants[5], onplants[6], palatal implants[7], zygoma ligatures[8], mini-plates[9] and mini-implants[10]. Mini-implants were proposed eighteen years ago and their use is now widespread in clinical practice. The main advantages of mini-implants are: small size, low cost, easy insertion and removal, with little discomfort to the patient, and the possibility of immediate load application[11-14].

Orthodontic mini-implants, also called miniscrews, microimplant, or orthodontic pins, are classified as temporary anchorage devices (TAD), since the main condition for their use is that osseointegration is not expected to occur, so these appliances can be removed on conclusion of treatment mechanics[15]. This is only possible due to the type of titanium alloy in the composition of most of the mini-implants: Ti-6AL-4V. This alloy has excellent surface characteristics, biocompatibility, mechanical strength and corrosion resistance[16], but it has lower bioactivity than the commercially pure titanium used to manufacture dental implants[17].

Since osseointegration is not required, immediate load[11-14] will be applied to the miniscrew, if stability is achieved after its insertion in bone tissue. Classically, stability can be divided into primary and secondary types. Primary stability is a mechanical parameter defined as the lack of mobility of the device in the bone bed after its insertion[18]. It depends on the close contact between the surface of the mini-

4

implant and the bone[19, 20]. On the other hand, secondary stability, also called late stability, occurs after healing[19]. Primary stability depends on the mini-implant design[21], insertion technique[21], and bone quality and quantity at the receptor site[21-24]. The term bone quality has not been clearly defined in the literature. It includes physiological and structural aspects and the degree of bone tissue mineralization[25]. Some bone properties, such as bone mineral density[26, 27] and cortical thickness[28-30] have been related to the stability of mini-implants and recent studies have suggested that both cortical[25, 27] and trabecular bone[27] play an important role.

Most of the failures occur immediately after mini-implant placement[31], probably due to insufficient primary stability, which causes poor healing and premature loss of the device[19]. If initial mechanical retention of the miniscrew is not observed, a larger screw should be used, or the insertion site should be changed[32]. On the other hand, exaggerated tension during insertion may result in heating and damage to the bone tissue[33], including ischemia and necrosis, or even fracture of the miniscrew[21].

As the aims of orthodontic treatment are: to achieve the best balance and harmony of facial lines; stability of dentures after treatment; efficient chewing mechanism and the maintenance of healthy mouth tissues[34]; the soft tissue surrounding miniscrew must be kept healthy. The surgical procedure of miniscrew insertion must be carefully performed to avoid damage to surrounding structures since miniscrews can be placed in various alveolar bone locations. Possible insertion sites in the maxilla are: the nasal spine (lower portion), palate, alveolar process, and the infra-zygomatic ridge. In the mandible, the areas of choice for the placement of mini-implants are the alveolar process, the retromolar area and the mandibular symphysis[17].

Careful operation can involve the use of a radiograph, CT, or surgical stent[35]. Nevertheless, complications can arise during miniscrew placement, such as trauma to the periodontal ligament, dental root or nerves, nasal and maxillary sinus perforation and subcutaneous air emphysema[36]. If the miniscrew comes into contact with the root during insertion, devitalization of the tooth is a possible consequence[37]. The friction of inserting a mini-implant into bone can initiate an inflammatory reaction, resulting in damages to the bone tissue[38, 39] or its active remodeling around the root, which can induce external root resorption or ankylosis[35]. Proximity to the root can also induce failure of the device[40].

Complications during orthodontic loading such as aphthous ulceration, soft-tissue coverage of the miniscrew head, soft tissue inflammation, infection, and peri-implantitis may also occur[36]. Auxiliaries attached between the screw head and the archwire (coil springs, elastomeric chains, hooks, and ligation wires) should be adjusted not to touch the gingiva or oral mucosa to prevent pain and discomfort, although damage to soft tissues is temporary in most cases[41].

Mini-implants are anatomically divided into the following parts: threads – the active portion that is inserted into the bone tissue; transmucosal neck – the region that remains in contact with the covering soft tissue; and head – the portion exposed to the mouth and used for applying orthodontic force by means of elastics, springs, power arms or ligatures. Each parameter with reference to the head, transmucosal collar and thread designs varies according to the miniscrew manufacturers, as shown in Figure1.

Geometric characteristics of miniscrews, such as shape, diameter, length, thread form and pitch, have an impact on primary stability[42]. However, no "optimal design" has yet been defined. Thread diameters may range from 1 to 2mm. The apical portion of the thread is narrower than its body to favor mini-implant insertion and minimize surgical trauma. Furthermore, this feature reduces the risk of root contact[17]. The thread cutting power is an important feature to consider in the choice of the device[43]. Self-drilling and self-tapping mini-implants present the following differences: while the self-drilling type has an extremely thin and sharp apex, it does not require the use of any additional bone drilling procedure in most cases; the self-tapping type has a rounded apex and requires a perforation made with a drill at the insertion site [44].

The diameter of the mini-implant should be chosen according to the insertion site, and the available space at it, verified by intraoral radiography or tomography. When a mini-implant is going to be inserted between the roots, a thinner diameter is recommended in order to reduce the risk of root contact. On the other hand, the fracture risk is related to the diameter of the mini-implant used[17]. Common sense and caution are recommended in such cases.

The transmucosal neck presents varying lengths, to enable it to fit into different thicknesses of soft tissue[45]. As the neck is the portion that remains in contact with the covering soft tissue, it must be well polished. The presence of irregularities helps colonization by microorganisms because they protect the bacteria from salivary flow cleaning power, chewing, swallowing and cleaning procedures, allowing the establishment of less reversible links between microorganisms in biofilm[46]. Plaque accumulation may cause problems such as acute or chronic inflammation, infection[47] and consequent loss of the device. The postoperative oral hygiene is another factor of great importance for the stability of the mini-implant. It is essential to guide the patient on the necessary measures to control biofilm. Some authors have recommended the use of chlorhexidine[36], but a recent study has shown that the mechanical cleaning of mini-implants maintains control of microorganisms around these devices [48].

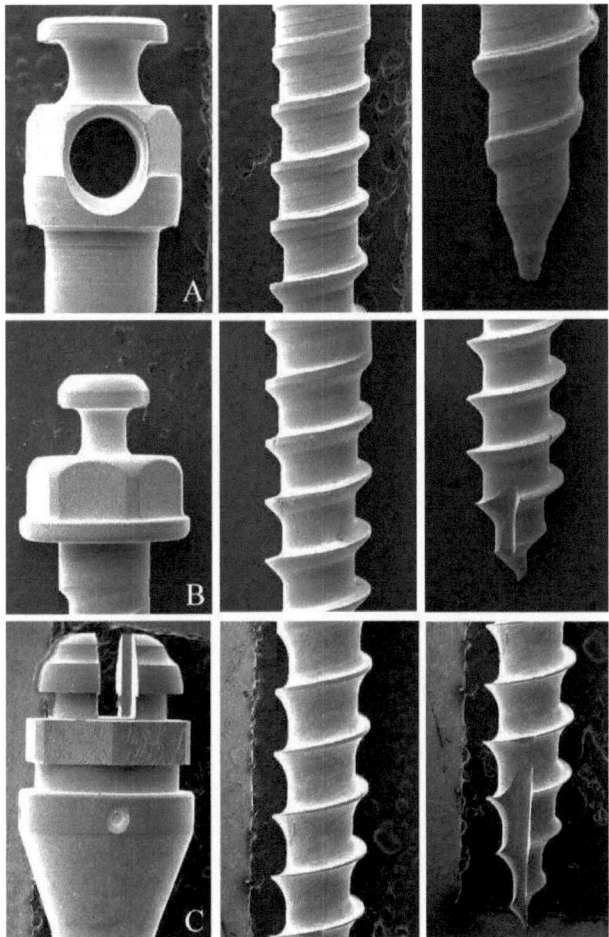

Figure 1: Orthodontic miniscrew systems visualized by Scanning electron microscopy (10 x magnifications) with details of the head, thread and tip. **A.** INP® system; **B.** RMO® Dual-Top; **C.** Tomas® system.

The head of the mini-implant also varies in anatomy and size depending on the purpose of the device (buttonlike or bracketlike) (Figure 2). Bigger or sharper heads can predispose to traumatic lesions to soft tissues (Figures 3 and 4), however, they do not appear to be a direct risk factor for miniscrew stability. Nevertheless, their presence might predict a higher level of soft tissue inflammation and make it difficult to control plaque.

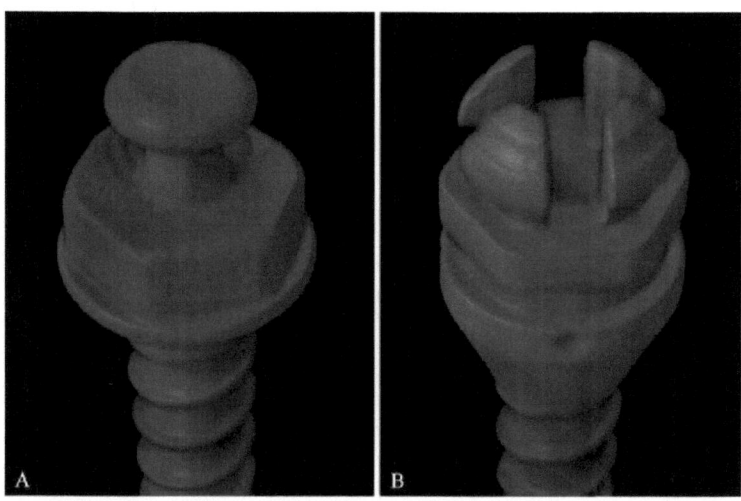

Figure 2: Micro-CT reconstructions of two samples of commercially available miniscrews. **A.** Buttonlike head design of RMO® Dual-Top (Rocky Mountain Orthodontics); **B.** Bracketlike head design of Tomas® system (Dentaurum GmbH & Co. KG).

The placement of a healing abutment, wax pellet, or a large elastic separator over the miniscrew head, with daily use of chlorhexidine (0.12%, 10 mL), typically prevents ulceration and improves patient comfort[36]. Covering the miniscrew head to prevent soft tissue damage has not been a routine procedure in Orthodontics until now, but it can be very useful, as seen in Marquezan *et al* (Figure 5)[49]. The mini-implant placed between the central incisors created ulceration in the frenulum 48 hours after insertion, in spite of having placed an elastic chain on its head. The solution was to insert a resin covering on the screw head to give the patient comfort. After four days, the tissue was healthy (Figure 5B). The use of dental wax might also help to reduce trauma and discomfort, but the wax is easily dislodged from the miniscrew head. In this case report, the light polymerized resin Bioplic (Biodinâmica, Ibiporã, Paraná, Brazil) was used.

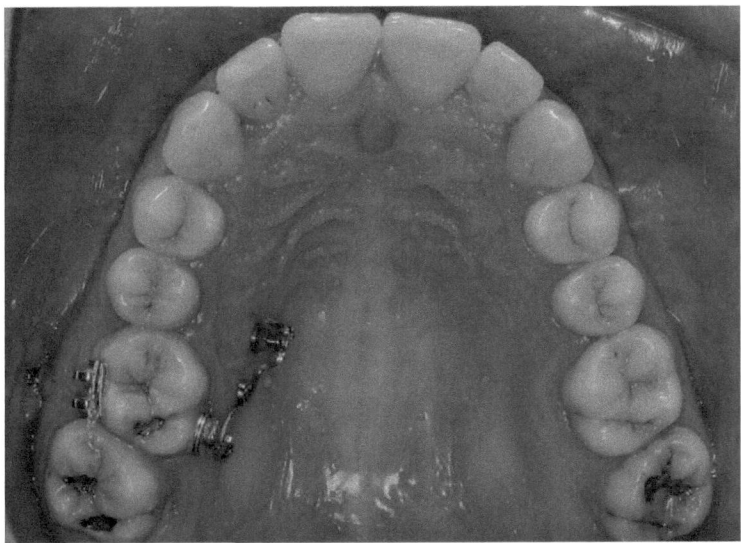

Figure 3: Orthodontic miniscrews were used for molar intrusion. The screw inserted on the buccal side caused ulceration in the jugal mucosa (blue arrow).

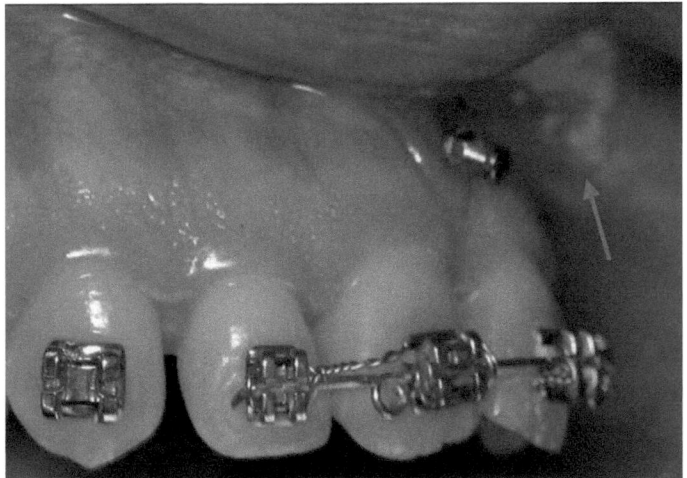

Figure 4: An orthodontic miniscrew was inserted between the maxillary central incisors for intrusion and caused ulceration in the upper lip (blue arrow).

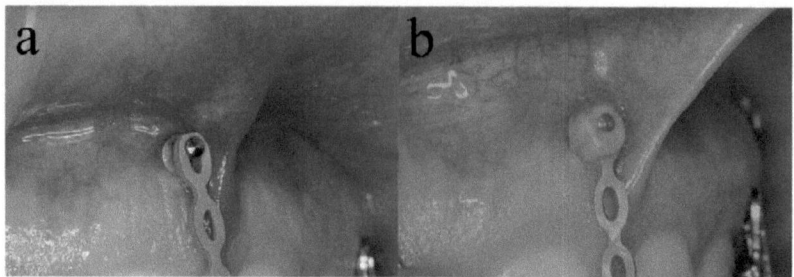

Figure 5: A. Traumatic lesion in the frenulum caused by a miniscrew; **B.** After the placement of resin to cover the head, the tissue healed in four days. *These images were extracted from Marquezan M, de Freitas AO, Nojima LI. Miniscrew covering: an alternative to prevent traumatic lesions. Am J Orthod Dentofacial Orthop 2012;141:242-244.*

Despite the last edition of classic textbooks such as "Orthodontics: Current Principles and Techniques" – written by Graber, Vanarsdall and Vig[50] – and "Contemporary Orthodontics" – written by Proffit, Fields and Sarver[51] – presented a chapter describing the use of miniscrews as anchorage devices, and contained illustrations of resins covering the miniscrew head, the use of resin covering is not emphasized.

In this book, two dental resins will be presented: Bioplic (Biodinâmica, Ibiporã, Paraná, Brazil) – the temporary resin cited above – and Top Comfort (FGM, Joinville, Santa Catarina, Brazil) – a resin bracket protector. Series of cases were treated in Orthodontic Department of Federal University of Rio de Janeiro (UFRJ), using these two resins to protect the mucosa and avoid patient discomfort, and presented good results. Considering that the use of dental resins for covering mini implants promotes their direct contact with oral soft tissues, the cytotoxicity of the resins was also tested.

2. A brief history of skeletal anchorage

The history of miniscrew development refers to several models of temporary skeletal devices designed for orthodontic anchorage in the last decades, with a great variety of materials, designs and insertion sites.

In 1945, Gainsforth and Higley described a method of basal bone anchorage, in which vitallium screws were placed in the mandibular ramus of six dogs to provide anchorage reinforcement for canine retraction. The use of vitallium was justified because of its wide use and acceptance in several types of bone surgeries at that time[52], however the vitallium screws failed in approximately 2 and 4 weeks. The results indicated the need for appliances with smaller diameters and less invasive surgical procedures in order to reduce the risks of infection and consequently, the screw loosening.

Two decades later, other materials were tested for manufacturing orthodontic implants. Vitreous carbon implants[53] and bioglass-coated ceramic implants[54] were compatible with bone, but they failed because none of them showed consistent long-term attachment of bone to the implant interface[55].

Clinical use of the vitallium screw was described in 1983 by Creekmore and Eklund, with the purpose of deep overbite correction[4]. The screw inserted in the nasal spine did not move during the application of the orthodontic force and the intrusion of maxillary incisors was successful. This was the first clinical report of skeletal anchorage in a human, and encouraged further investigations concerning the clinical use of the skeletal anchorage[4].

In the same period, other system of skeletal anchorage was proposed representing a superior type of rigid anchorage devices, due to the osseointegration process: the dental implants[56, 57]. Osseointegration was defined by Brånemark (1983)[58] as the direct contact between living bone and the surface of a load-carrying implant at the histological level. Clinically, it is a biomechanical phenomenon whereby asymptomatic rigid fixation of the implant is achieved and maintained in bone during functional loading[59]. Roberts *et al* stated that it was necessary to wait a period of 4 to 5 months for osseointegration, prior to the application of orthodontic force to the dental implant[56, 57]. Considering the increase in treatment time and higher financial costs of this type of treatment approach, it should be considered an option for orthodontic purposes only in cases in which it would be used in a prosthetic treatment plan simultaneously[60].

The osseointegration process was also applied to the onplant, a device proposed by Block and Hoffman in 1995[6] (Figure 6). It was a titanium alloy disk (2mm high and 10mm Ø) with a hydroxyapatite surface. Onplants differed from implants since the insertion was subperiosteal, so that they adhered only to the outer surface of the bone[61]. Its anatomy was favorable for palatal insertion; so this device was not limited to edentulous areas[6]. After its insertion, it was necessary to wait a 10-week healing period before surgically exposing the onplant and attaching a ball-shaped abutment to it. This was subsequently connected to orthodontic bands on the maxillary molar teeth by a transpalatal arch. This mechanism has been shown to resist continuous orthodontic force of over 300 g, which is comparable to the force required for conventional space closure of orthodontic extraction sites. However, the lack of primary stability and the need for a period of waiting were considered disadvantages[60]. After correction of the malocclusion, the onplant should be removed using an osteotome. The authors did not elaborate on any complications associated with this procedure[55], but defects caused by the removal as a result of the osteointegration have been reported [62].

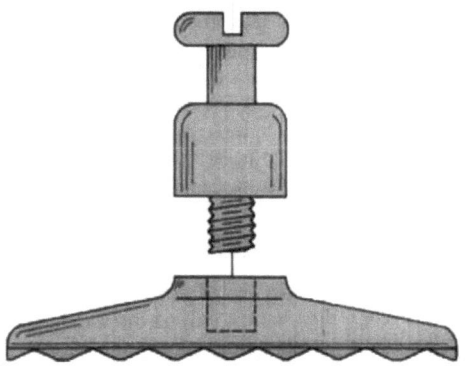

Figure 6: Diagram of Onplant. The lower portion of the device was a titanium alloy disk with a hydroxyapatite surface. The upper portion was the abutment used to connect to the transpalatal arch. *This image was extracted from Wehrbein H, Merz BR, Diedrich P, Glatzmaier J. The use of palatal implants for orthodontic anchorage. Design and clinical application of the orthosystem. Clin Oral Implants Res 1996;7(4):410-6.*

In 1996, Wehrbein *et al*[7] described the Orthosystem (Institute Straumann, Waldenburg, Switzerland), an endosseous orthodontic implant anchor system for palatal anchorage. The titanium devices were 3.3 mm in diameter, and were composed of a screw-type endosseous section of between 4 mm and 6 mm in length (depending on palatal depth), a cylindrical transmucosal neck, and an abutment, to which a transpalatal arch was attached (Figure 7)[55]. The anterior midsagittal area of the palate was the placement site for these implants. It was necessary to wait 3 months for healing prior to orthodontic loading[61]. To maximize stability, the implant had a sandblasted acid-etched surface, which resulted in a high level of direct bone contact[55].

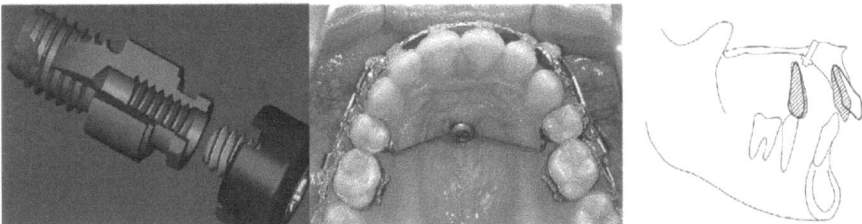

Figure 7: The Orthosystem implant. **A.** Diagram of the palatal implant; **B.** Clinical application for anterior retraction: see the transpalatal arch attached on palatal implant; **C.** Cephalogram showing movement of the incisors and premolar stability. See the insertion place of the implant in the anterior portion of the palate. *These images were extracted from Wehrbein H, Merz BR, Diedrich P, Glatzmaier J. The use of palatal implants for orthodontic anchorage. Design and clinical application of the orthosystem. Clin Oral Implants Res 1996;7(4):410-6.*

Both Onplant and palatal implants (Orthosystem) did not find widespread acceptance into clinical routine, because of the long waiting period before application of loading forces (for osseointegration), which added significantly to the treatment time, made it difficult to remove them after treatment, and high costs.

In 1997, Kanomi[10] described a mini-implant, which was developed from a mini-bone screw used for fixing bone plates. The mini-implant was successfully used for mandibular incisor intrusion and correction of curve of Spee. Within 4 months, the incisors had been intruded 6 mm. Although its insertion required flap opening, and it was necessary to wait for osseointegration, it was nevertheless considered the first miniscrew used in Orthodontics (Figure 8).

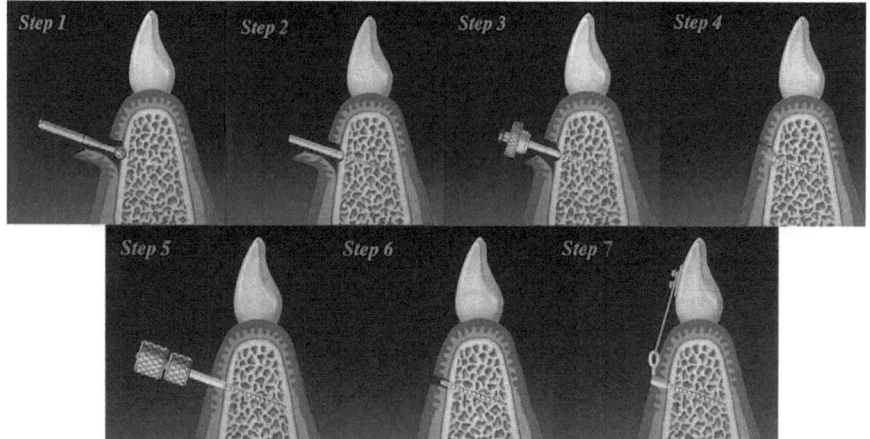

Figure 8: Diagram showing the insertion technique of the first mini-implant proposed by Kanomi (1997). First, a mucoperiosteal flap is reflected for cortical perforation, using a round bur (Step 1). After this, a pilot drill with the same length as that of the mini-implant should be used (Step 2) prior to its insertion with a screwdriver (Step 3). Then, the mini-implant is sutured over for osseointegration (Step 4). After this period, the gingival tissue should be exposed (Steps 5 and 6) and a titanium bone plate attached to the head of mini-implant, and tied to the bracket with ligature wire (Step 7). *These images were extracted from Kanomi R. Mini-implant for orthodontic anchorage. J Clin Orthod 1997;31(11):763-7.*

A year later, Costa *el al* (1998) developed miniscrews especially designed for orthodontic anchorage. The titanium miniscrew had a special bracket-like head that could be used for either direct or indirect anchorage. The screws were placed manually with a screwdriver directly through the mucosa, without a flap, and were loaded immediately. In contrast to osseointegrated implants, these devices were smaller in diameter, had smoother surfaces, and were designed to be loaded shortly after placement[61].

The concept of using basal bones for skeletal anchorage resurfaced in the 1990s. Melsen (1998) described the use of zygoma ligatures[8]. Steel ligatures (0.012") were inserted into the zygomatic bone of partially edentulous patients for intrusion and retraction of maxillary incisors. A portion of the ligatures was exposed to the oral environment for activation of nickel-titanium springs.

In the following year, Umemori *et al* (1999)[9] introduced a skeletal anchorage system (SAS) with titanium mini-plates. Two cases of severe open-bite malocclusion were treated with the use of mini-plates inserted in the apical regions of mandibular molars bilaterally. The intrusion movement was successfully achieved by using elastic forces applied to mini-plates.

From the time the above-mentioned devices were introduced, up to the present days, mini-implants and mini-plates have been very useful[63, 64], and are often called temporary anchorage devices (TADs)[65]. The mini-plates bolted to the basal bone, do not interfere in the path of the tooth to be moved, allow the application of greater forces[66] and present failure rates ranging from 3%[67] to 7.3%[68]. These are considered ideal characteristics for orthopedic treatments, since these systems could effectively be applied for growth modification purposes other than for tooth movement only.[69] On the other hand, mini-plate placement and removal require two surgical procedures, involving flap incision, reflection, and closure, possibly causing fear of pain in the patient[70]. Mini-implants present versatility, easy insertion and removal, good healing, possibility of early loading and reduced financial costs. These characteristics are responsible for the higher demand of these devices in the orthodontic field[15, 71, 72].

Using TADs, orthodontists can now perform a variety of tooth movements such as: (1) retract and realign anterior teeth without posterior support, (2) close edentulous spaces in first-molar extraction sites, (3) correct midlines in patients with missing posterior teeth, (4) re-establish proper transverse anteroposterior positions of isolated molar abutments, (5) intrude or extrude teeth, (6) protract or retract an arch; and it is also possible to apply orthopedic traction[55].

After eighteen years from the time they were first proposed[10], orthodontic mini-implants continue to be an extensively discussed issue in scientific research. Several studies have been conducted with the purpose of investigating factors associated with miniscrew stability, especially motivated by the current success rates ranging from approximately 80% to 83.6%[68, 73, 74]. Several possible causes for miniscrew failures have been proposed, such as: patient age[29], mandibular plane angle[31], the insertion site characteristics (of the adjacent hard and soft tissues)[33, 40, 75-77], inflammation of peri-implant tissues[31, 33], factors related to the mini-implant (such as type and dimensions)[31, 76], quantity of insertion torque[29, 78, 79] and levels of forces exerted[76, 80].

It is known that the success rate of miniscrews is related to their primary stability, which is influenced by the host bone properties, surgical insertion techniques, and the miniscrew geometric characteristics[21, 81-86]. Further investigation is being conducted as regards factors involved in the periods of healing of the mini-implants in humans. Considering both mechanical and biological assessment, it has been observed that the degree of stability as well as the levels of inflammatory mediators varied throughout the healing period[87-90].

3. Patients' perception of miniscrews as anchorage devices

Patients often feel pain during orthodontic treatment, for example during tooth separation, initial archwire insertion and debonding[91, 92]. In a study conducted by Kvam et al (1989)[93], 38% of patients said that activation of the appliance caused the most discomfort. The pain after activation lasted for only 2–3 days (71%), but 20% had pain for longer than 3 days. In this study, the authors also evaluated ulceration frequency caused by orthodontic devices. Only four patients had never had oral ulceration during treatment, and 47% of the patients said that ulcers caused by the fixed appliance were the most annoying part of the treatment.

In spite of mini-implants having been introduced in the market in the 1990s, few studies have focused on the patients' experience relative to their expectations, acceptance and preferences during treatment with miniscrews[91]. Little is known about the pain and discomfort caused by miniscrews[91, 92] and there are few investigations into the oral ulceration they cause[49].

Reynders et al (2009)[94] performed a systematic review to evaluate success and complications related to the use of miniscrews. Inflammation, discomfort and pain were adverse effects described for these devices. The majority of the articles included in the review did not evaluate these outcomes. The results of the articles are described below. Freudenthaler et al (2001)[23] and Chaddad et al (2008)[95] reported minor pain after placement, which lasted only 1 day in a few of the patients of the sample. Kuroda et al (2007)[96] analyzed both the quality and duration of pain during the first 2 weeks after placement, comparing a flap and flapless group. One hour after implantation, 95% of the patients who had screws placed after raising a mucoperiosteal flap reported pain, compared with 50% of those who had undergone a flapless procedure. After 2 weeks, the values were 10% and 0% for the respective techniques. A similar finding was recorded by Miyawaki et al (2003)[31], who found more pain in patients of the flap group than those in the flapless group within a week after implant placement.

Baxmann et al (2010)[92] evaluated the pain and discomfort experienced by orthodontic patients by comparing how they rated pain associated with miniscrew placement, tooth extraction, and gingival tissue removal in preparation for implant placement. Fifty-six miniscrews were placed in 28 consecutive orthodontic patients for anchorage reinforcement in the maxilla for an en-masse retraction. For all patients, extractions of maxillary, or maxillary and mandibular premolars had been planned. The recruited patients were randomized into 2 groups according to the timing of the extractions. In group A, at least 1 extraction was performed before miniscrew placement. In group B, all extractions were performed after placement of the miniscrew. Furthermore, all patients had 2 different surgical procedures for placement. On 1 side, the gingival tissue was removed before placement. On the contralateral side, the implant was placed transgingivally. Each patient's perception of pain and discomfort was evaluated by a questionnaire before, immediately after, and 1 week after the intervention. The discomfort experienced during the extractions was described as very painful by 50% of the patients. Pain and discomfort were significantly more severe than during tissue removal and miniscrew placement (P<0.05). Minisccrew placement produced no pain in 30% of the patients and was described as the least painful procedure (P<0.05). Transgingival miniscrew placement was significantly preferred by all patients (P<0.05).

Lehnen et al (2011)[91, 97] evaluated the patient's perception on insertion and removal of miniscrews. The word 'pin' was used rather than microimplant, mini-implant or miniscrew. By using a less threatening term, it was hoped to minimize patient apprehension[91, 97]. For the first study[91], the insertion of the mini-implants was evaluated. A total of 30 patients undergoing orthodontic treatment with mini-implants to reinforce skeletal anchorage were enrolled and randomly divided into two groups, A and B. Two different insertion techniques and two different anesthesia injection methods were used. In group A, pre-drilling was carried out using a dental handpiece so that the pins could then be inserted manually. In group B, a completely manual placement method was used for the pins by means of self-cutting implants. All implants were inserted in the interradicular area of the maxillary second premolar and maxillary first molars in both maxillary quadrants and Tomas® pins were used in all patients (length: 8.0 mm, diameter: 1.6 mm; Dentaurum, Ispringen, Germany). It was found that it made no difference to the patients whether the orthodontist drilled before implant insertion or whether a self-drilling implant was used. The patients found the noise from the dental handpiece more unpleasant than the pain, and as regards the self-drilling implants, the pressure was more unpleasant than the pain. Considering the anesthesia method, patients preferred injections directly into the area where the implants were to be inserted. Their reasons for this were the shorter period of numbness after treatment and potentially quicker therapy. Using this method it was possible to place the implants just seconds after the injection, whereas a 3-min wait was necessary using the standard infiltration technique. The patients found this delay more important than the pain intensity during the injection itself.

In the second study[97], removal of the miniscrews was evaluated. Twenty-five patients were randomly assigned to Group A or Group B. In Group A, the miniscrews were removed with a handpiece, while in the Group B patients' miniscrews were removed completely by hand. In addition, all patients received an injection of local anesthetic into one half of the jaw. No anesthetic was used in the other half of the jaw. When the patients were asked about their pain perception, it was demonstrated that the injection itself caused more pain than the actual surgery ($p<0.005$). Moreover, miniscrew removal using the handpiece led to significantly more discomfort, due to the noise associated with its use rather than from the actual pain itself[97].

All of the studies cited above focused on patient perception of pain and discomfort related to the surgical procedure. However, from an evidence-based point of view, there is also a need for studies concerning patient acceptance of these new approaches from a long term perspective[98].

Feldmann *et al* (2012)[98] performed a clinical trial to evaluate and compare perceived pain, discomfort, and jaw function impairment between orthodontic treatments combined with skeletal anchorage and treatment using conventional anchorage with headgear or transpalatal bar. Patient perception was evaluated from baseline to the retention phase. A total of 120 adolescent patients about to start orthodontic treatment were randomized into three groups with different anchorage: A – underwent installation of a skeletal anchorage in palate (Onplant or Orthosystem implant); B – received headgear; C – a transpalatal bar. Questionnaires were used to assess pain intensity, discomfort, analgesic consumption, and jaw function impairment. Pain scores overall peaked on day 2 and was almost back to baseline on day 7. There was no significant differences in perceived pain intensity between the three anchorage groups, and there was no difference in the use of analgesics. Pain intensity from the palate and tongue was significantly higher in the skeletal anchorage and transpalatal bar groups compared with the headgear group. This in combination with more discomfort in form of soreness was probably an effect of the inconvenience with palatal appliances. However, this did not affect the patients' eating habits and speech. Median values for pain intensity and discomfort were comparatively moderate, but some patients described it as the worst imaginable. It is well known that perception of pain is subjective, with no or little relationship between the objective strength of a pain stimulus. The results confirmed that there were very few significant differences between patients' perceptions of skeletal and conventional anchorage systems during orthodontic treatment.

Zawawi (2014)[99] studied the patients' acceptance, expectation, and experience of pain with orthodontic temporary miniscrews. Questionnaires were distributed to 165 orthodontic patients (or their parents), with a mean age of 21.4 (±4.1) years, who were candidates for miniscrew insertion. Using the numerical rating scale, patients who received miniscrews as part of their orthodontic treatment were also asked to rate the pain or discomfort experience after miniscrew placement. Although only 12.7% had heard about miniscrews, 82.4% agreed to have miniscrews placed to facilitate orthodontic tooth movement. Eighty-three subjects who needed miniscrews as part of their orthodontic treatment completed two more sets of questions at 6 and 24 hours after miniscrew insertion. Thirty two percent did not require any pain medication postplacement, while 59.1% required a single dose and only 8.4% required two doses. A total of 76 patients (91.6%) said that they would recommend this procedure. The author concluded that patients did accept the miniscrew as a treatment option in orthodontics, preferred miniscrews to extractions, and postoperative pain was significantly low.

There is still a gap on literature concerning patients' perception of the use of miniscrews in buccal alveolar bone, when comparing miniscrew head anatomy, mechanics applied and head coverage or not.

4.   *Dental resins used to cover the miniscrews head*

It is desirable for a resin used to cover miniscrews to be easily inserted and removed, and to present no toxicity to the surrounding tissues. Thinking of the ease of insertion and removal, professors and post-graduate students of our Dental School (Federal University of Rio de Janeiro) started using temporary resins – Bioplic (Biodinâmica, Ibiporã, Paraná, Brazil) and Top Comfort (FGM, Joinville, Santa Catarina, Brazil) – for miniscrew head covering in the clinics of the institution. Both temporary resins present some elasticity after light polymerization, so they can be removed using a dental probe. Some clinicians use composite resin, however, burs are required to remove it (Figure 9).

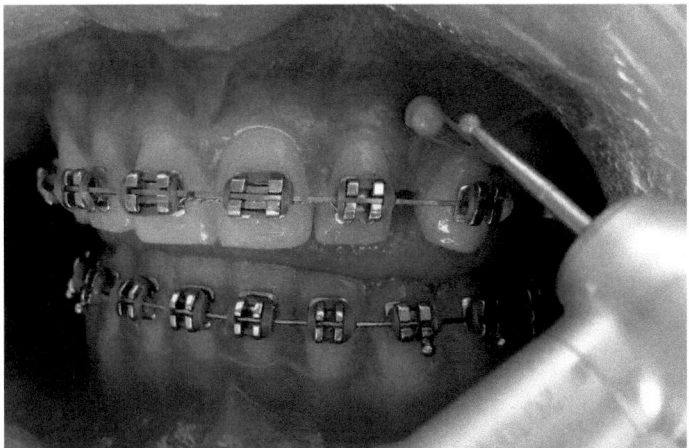

Figure 9: Composite resin (Transbond XT, 3M Unitek, Monrovia, Calif, USA) used to cover the miniscrew head. A bur is needed for its removal.

Bioplic is a resin material that acquires a hardened rubber-consistency after light polymerization. It is used to temporarily seal cavities, as well as the screw on the implant, forming a mechanical barrier to isolate the screw from contact with the oral cavity fluids, and to protect patient from orthodontic devices that can injure soft tissues (Figure 10).

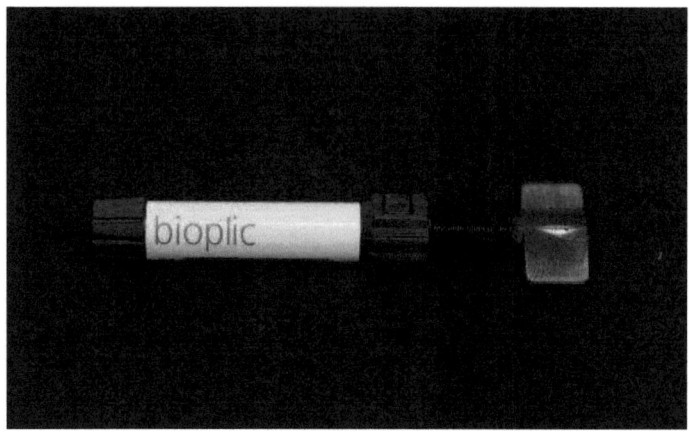

Figure 10: Commercial presentation of Bioplic.

The placement technique of this resin is simple and fast. Relative isolation is required and it is necessary to dry the miniscrew head (Figure 11A). Using a tooth sculpture tool (or any other similar instrument), the filling material can easily be shaped (Figure 11B). After this, light polymerization must be performed for 40 seconds (Figure 11C and D). In the next appointment, a probe can be inserted at the junction between material and implant to remove the material (Figure 11E).

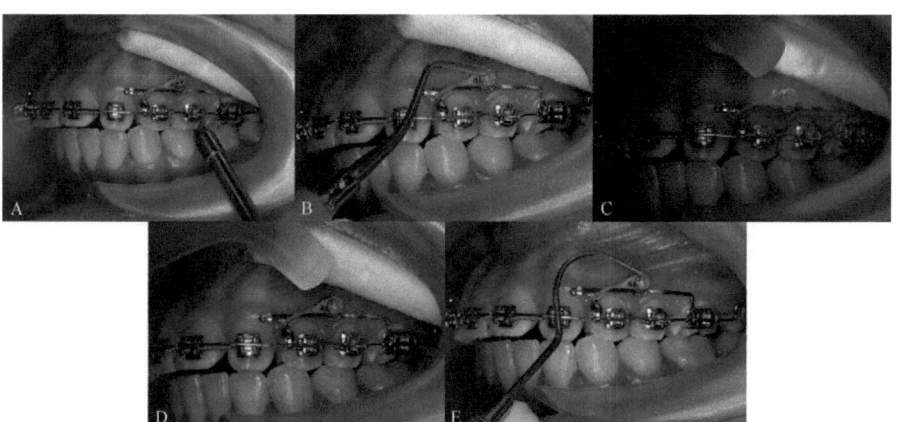

Figure 11: Placement technique for Bioplic. A. drying miniscrew head; B. application of the material; C. light polymerization (40 seconds); D. aspect of the resin after polymerization; E. removal of the resin with a probe.

There are many other light polymerizable temporary fillings available on the market, which remain semi-flexible after polymerization, and they might be good covering materials for mini implant heads, such as ProvimasterF (Wilcos, Petrópolis, Rio de Janeiro, Brazil), ClipF (Voco, Cuxhaven, Germany), First Fill (Pentron Clinical Technologies, Wallingford CT, USA) and Soleil (DMG America LLC, Englewood, NJ, USA).

In 2013, another alternative was launched in this field: Top Comfort (FGM, Joinville, Santa Catarina, Brazil), which is a light polymerized resin bracket protector for professional application. It was designed to prevent eventual injuries caused by the contact of sharp orthodontic devices, such as brackets, tubes, jigs and miniscrews with the patient's oral soft tissues. It is a fluid resin supplied in a tube with tip that facilitates insertion (Figure 12).

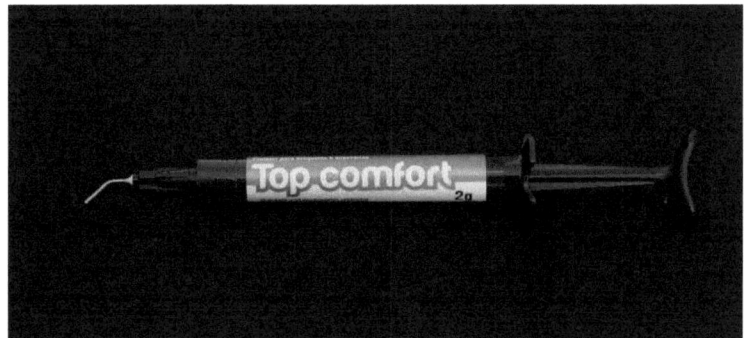

Figure 12: Commercial presentation of Top Comfort.

Its application requires relative isolation, and the mini-implant head must be dried with compressed air (Figure 13A). After drying, the resin can be applied on miniscrew head, without need of a sculpture tool. In its fluid phase, the resin is milky-colored (Figure 13B). Next, the resin must be light polymerized for 30 seconds (Figure 13C), and assumes a translucent appearance (Figure 13D). It is recommended to use a light-curing appliance of over 400 mW/cm2. As with Bioplic, a probe can be used to remove the material when necessary (Figure 13E).

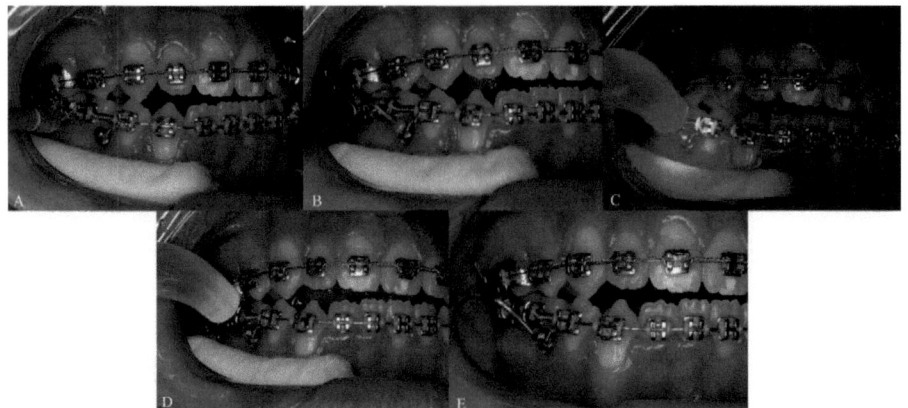

Figure 13: Placement technique for Top Comfort. **A.** drying miniscrew head; **B.** application of the material; **C.** light polymerization (20 seconds); **D.** aspect of the resin after curing; **E.** removal of the resin with a probe.

Biofilm can grow and establish itself on several types of surfaces, such as living tissues, teeth, orthodontic accessories, resins and implants[100]. The importance of a polished transmucosal neck and patients' education to perform adequate biofilm control around the miniscrew to prevent inflammation and subsequent miniscrew loss was previously emphasized in Chapter 1. The peri-implant area determined by the gingival attachment to the neck of the implant, which is responsible for mucosal seal and protection of mini-implant health, should be resistant to bacterial adhesion and retention[48]. Rougher surfaces favor greater plaque accumulation and retention[46], because they increase the area available for colonization. The presence of pits and grooves also protects bacteria from removal forces[101]. When applying resin covering on a miniscrew head, care must be redoubled, because the resins may present porosities and they are not polished after placement. Their roughness may favor bacterial accumulation if the patient does not perform proper hygiene. Four methods of hygiene for mini-implants were tested *in vivo* by Osório[48]: mechanical hygiene, or mechanical hygiene associated with a chemical agent – chlorhexidine 0.12%, Triclosan 0.03%, or cetylpyridinium chloride 0.05%. The evaluation showed that microbial control is achieved by mechanical cleaning of the devices, without additional chemical agents.

When using both Bioplic and Top Comfort to cover the miniscrew head in patients at the Federal University of Rio de Janeiro, plaque accumulation and soft tissue inflammation around the miniscrew was observed in a few cases, usually associated with poor biofilm control in the whole mouth. These patients received extra hygiene instructions and professional cleaning afterwards. No sensitivity or allergic reactions were observed. Nevertheless, a study was conducted by our research group to evaluate the cytotoxicity of resins used for covering miniscrews (see the next chapter).

5.   Cytotoxicity assessment of the coverage resins

The use of light polymerized resins for covering mini implants promotes their direct contact with oral soft tissues and their use should be avoided if patients present sensitivity to any of the components of the formula[49]. According to Shehata *et al* (2013)[102], the majority of resin matrices consist of a mixture of various methacrylate monomers, such as bis-phenol-A-glycidyl dimethacrylate (BisGMA) and urethane dimethacrylate (UDMA) in combination with lower viscosity co-monomers such as, triethyleneglycol dimethacrylate (TEGDMA), tetraethyleneglycol dimethacrylate (TEEGDMA), ethyleneglycol dimethacrylate (EGDMA), neopentylglycol dimethacrylate (Neopen) or diethyleneglycol dimethacrylate (DEGDMA). They are released into the oral cavity through incomplete polymerization or degradation processes[102, 103]. The monomers released may induce local and systemic reactions in patients[104], causing epithelial proliferation, liquenoid reactions[105], hypersensitivity and allergic reactions[105-107].

Although several studies have been conducted with orthodontic adhesives,[108-110] there has been little emphasis with respect to the biocompatibility of temporary composites used for covering miniscrews. Therefore, our research group decided to test the temporary resins used in our Dental School.

5.1   Sample

Self-drilling miniscrews (Ti-6Al-4V alloy, 1.4 mm X 6 mm) (Sistema INP®, São Paulo, Brazil) and the two light polymerizing temporary resins, used in our Dental School for covering of orthodontic miniscrews - Bioplic (Biodinâmica, Ibiporã, Paraná, Brazil) and Top Comfort (FGM, Joinville, Santa Catarina, Brazil) (Table 1) - were selected for assessment of their cytotoxicity.

The experimental groups were divided based on the evaluation conditions: as-received from the manufacturer and after polymerization (isolated or associated with the miniscrew head). Therefore, 7 groups with 3 samples each were assessed as follows: group A – miniscrew (MS); group B – Bioplic as received; group C – Bioplic light-polymerized; group D – Bioplic + MS; group E – Top comfort as received; group F – Top comfort light-polymerized and group G – Top comfort + MS (Table 2). As the test was carried out in triplicate, in total there were 9 values for each group. All the miniscrews and resins used in the study were in sealed packages and obtained from the same product lot.

Table 1 Composition of the resins tested with their respective manufacturers and manufacturing lot.

Resin	Manufacture	Composition	Lot
Bioplic	Biodinâmica, Ibiporã, Paraná, Brazil	bis-GMA,[III] dymethacrylate groups (40%); organic filler (25.18%); silicium dioxide, catalysts and sodium fluoride.	706/14
Top comfort	FGM, Joinville, Santa Catarina, Brazil	Methacrylic monomers (as bis-EMA, TEGDMA and UDMA), stabilizer, camphorquinone, co-initiator, pigments and inorganic fillers (40%) of boro-aluminium-silicate and silica nanoparticulate.	270813

Table 2 Design of the experimental groups.

Group	Characteristics
A	Miniscrew (MS)
B	Bioplic as-received
C	Bioplic after light-polymerization
D	Bioplic after light- polymerization placed on MS head
E	Top comfort resin as-received
F	Top comfort after light- polymerization
G	Top comfort after light- polymerization placed on MS head

5.2 Sample preparation

The materials used were previously sterilized in an autoclave and with ultra-violet light exposure for 1 hour. A tooth sculpture tool was used to remove Bioplic resin due to its higher viscosity and consistency. However, the fluid nature of the Top comfort resin made it necessary for the material to be transferred from the tip of the material tube to a tooth probe. With this technique, it was possible to remove similar quantities of both materials.

The light polymerization (DB 685 – Dabi Atlante, Ribeirão Preto, SP, Brazil) of Bioplic lasted 40 seconds and Top Comfort 30 seconds, according to the manufacturer's instructions. The groups C and F were light polymerized on the tooth tools, while in the groups D and G, the light polymerization was performed after the resins were applied to the head portion of miniscrews (Figure 14).

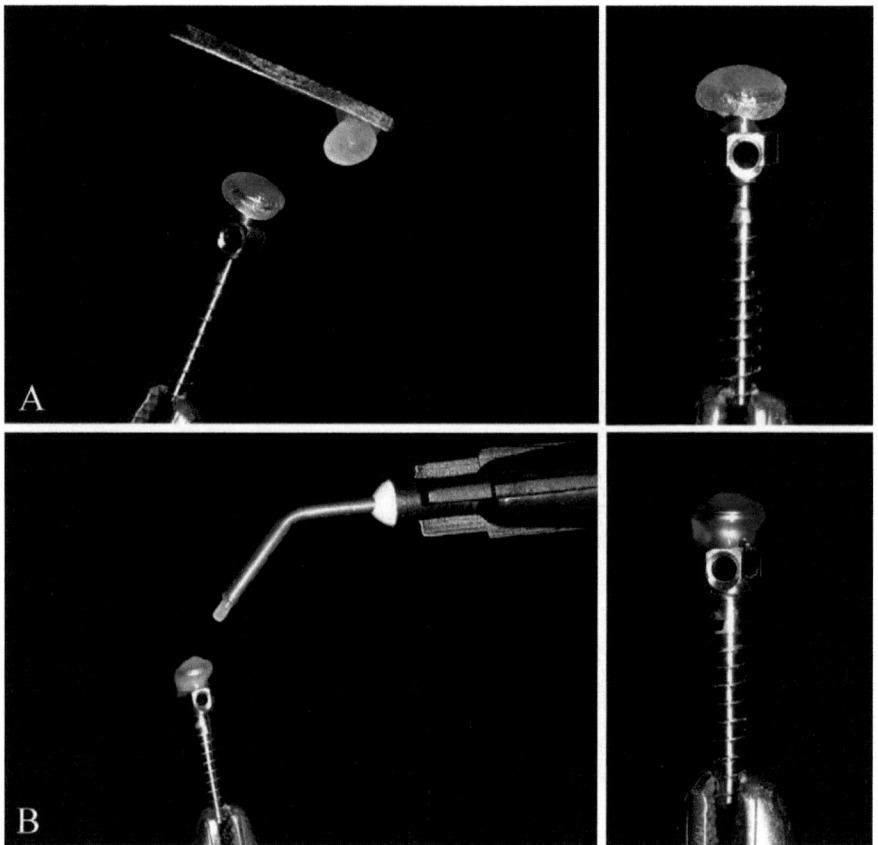

Figure 14: Aspect of as received and light-polymerized temporary fillings placed on MS head. **A.** Bioplic; **B.** Top comfort.

After preparation, all the samples were transferred to a 24-well plate containing Eagle's minimum essential medium (MEM) for cytotoxic evaluation (Figure 15).

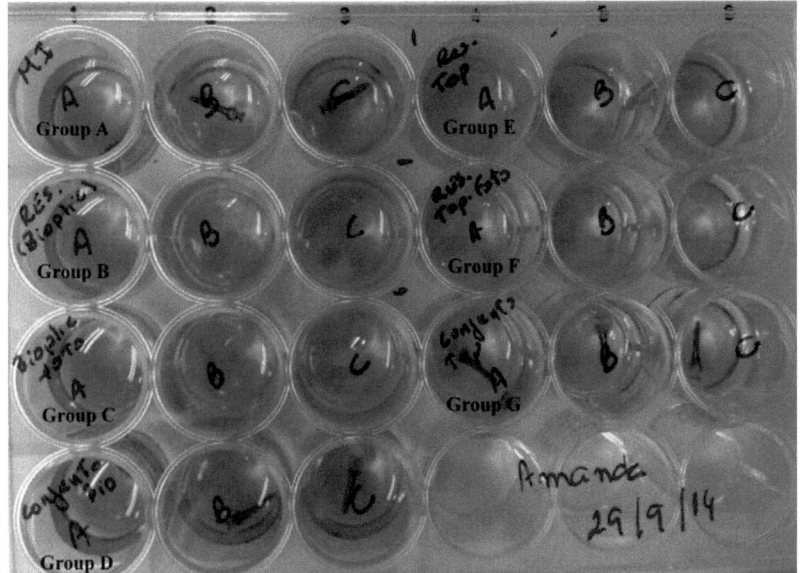

Figure 15: Experiment samples immersed in 1mL of MEM.

5.3   Cell Culture

Mouse lineage cells of L929 fibroblasts (American Type Culture Collection -
ATCC, Rockville, MD, USA) were cultivated in MEM (Cultilab, Campinas, Brazil)
with 2 mM of L-glutamine (Sigma, St.Louis, Missouri, USA), 50 μg/mL of
gentamicin (Schering Plough, Kenilworth, New Jersey, USA), 2.5 μg/mL of
fungizone (Bristol-Myers-Squib, New York, USA), 0.25 mM of sodium bicarbonate
solution (Merck, Darmstadt, Germany), 10 mM of HEPES (Sigma, St. Louis,
Missouri, USA), and 10% of foetal bovine serum (FBS) (Cultilab, Campinas, SP,
Brazil). After this, the cell culture medium was incubated at 37°C in a 5% CO_2
atmosphere for 24 hours.

5.4   Cytotoxicity assessment

The MEM was replaced with fresh medium every 24 hours. At time intervals
of 0, 24, 48, 72 hours, 7, 14 and 21 days the supernatants were collected in triplicate
for the analysis of toxicity to L929 cells. For each assessment, the supernatants were
transferred to 96-well plates with a single layer of L929 cells and maintained at 37 °C
in 5% CO_2 environment for 24 hours. In order to examine reaction of cells to extreme
conditions, two extra groups were included: Group H (positive control) constituted of

cells in contact with Tween 20 (Polyoxyethylenesorbitan monolaurate) and Group I (cell control), represented by cells not exposed to any of the materials tested.

On completion of the incubation period, the L929 cells were examined using an inverted microscope (E600 Nikon Eclipse, Japan). Morphologic evaluation and cell viability were determined using the method based on live cells incorporation of neutral-red dye described by Borenfreund and Puerner[112]. After a 24-hour incubation period, 100 µl of 0.01% neutral-red staining solution (Sigma™, St. Louis, Missouri, USA) was incorporated into the medium of each well, except for Group H (positive control), which had 100 µl of its medium replaced by 100 µl of Tween 20 before the neutral-red deposition. Next, the plate was maintained at 37°C for 3 hours to allow the incorporation of the dye into the living cells. After this, the wells were washed with 200 µl of PBS (130 mM NaCl; 2 mM KCl; 6 mM Na2HPO4 2H2O; 1 mM K2HPO4, pH = 7.2) and fixed for 5 minutes with 100 µl of 4% formaldehyde solution (Reagen™, Rio de Janeiro, Brazil), also in PBS. Finally, the dye was removed by adding 100 µl of 1% acetic acid solution (Vetec, Rio de Janeiro, Brazil) with 50% methanol (Reagen™, Rio de Janeiro, Brazil) to the medium. After 20 minutes, the optical density was measured with a spectrophotometer (BioTek™, Winooski, Vermont, USA) at a wavelength of 492 nm (μ=492 nm). The differences between the groups were visibly noticeable due to the color variation. The higher the level of the color shade (dye uptake), the greater the rate of viable cells as a result of lower toxic potential of the material (Figure 16). The cell viability (in percentage) was calculated considering the ratio between the optical density of the group tested and the optical density of the cell control group (assuming that the cell control group is equivalent to 100% of viable cells).

5.5   Statistical Analysis

Data were assessed with the software SPSS (version 17, SPSS Inc., USA). The normality and homogeneity of variables were verified by Kolmogorov-Smirnov and Levene's tests and intergroup comparisons were performed by ANOVA/ Tukey post-hoc tests. The level of significance adopted was 5%.

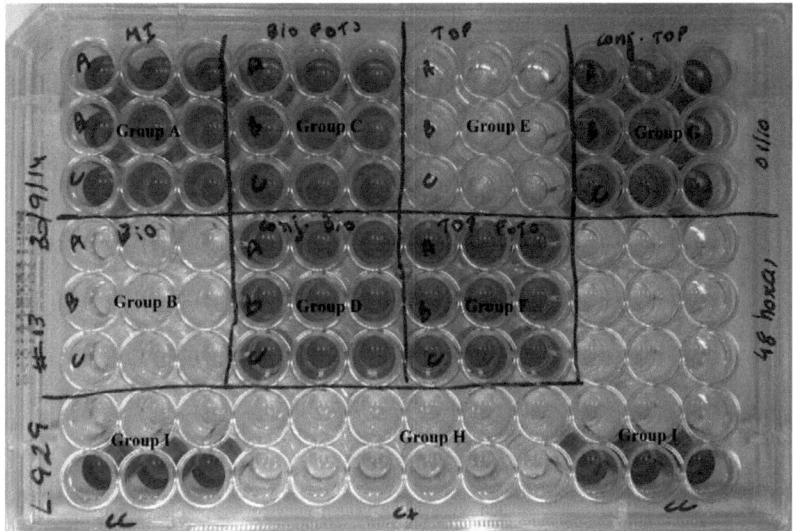

Figure 16: At 48 hours, a 96-well plate after the incorporation of the dye into the L929 cells.

5.6 Results and discussion

The morphological evaluation of the extreme groups, showed that in Group I the majority of spindle-shaped cells corresponded to fibroblasts in normal development. Whereas, in Group H, the presence of rounded and granular cells indicated an environment of cellular apoptosis. Depending on the cytotoxicity level, all of the other groups presented the same pattern as the above-mentioned groups. The results of quantitative intergroup comparisons for the experimental groups are given in Table 3 and Figure 17. Significant differences were found between the experimental and control groups, for all of the time intervals assessed (P<0.05).

The cell viability for the isolated miniscrew group ranged between 76.39% and 112.42%. In spite of the values at 24h, 48h, 14 and 21 days being slightly reduced in comparison with the cell control group, they were statistically different (P<0.05).

Both of the resins assessed as-received from the manufacturer (groups B and E), were extremely toxic until the last time interval of the study (P<0.05), presenting values equal to or even lower than those of the positive control group. At 24h, groups B (0.065±0.003), C (0.082±0.007), D (0.079±0.006), E (0.071±0.002) and G (0.178±0.030) exhibited severe toxicity and Group F (0.356±0.135) a moderate toxic activity (cell control: 0.703±0.053). A potential toxic activity was identified for Top Comfort resin until one week of the experiment.

31

TEGDMA is considered an important co-monomer present in the matrices of dental resins because it decreases their viscosity[109], however, a cytotoxic effect has been associated with this substance.[113, 114] We suppose that the flow consistency of Top Comfort resin, as well as its prolonged cytotoxic effect at the time intervals of 48h, 72h and 7 days, might be explained by the presence of TEGDMA in its matrix. It should be highlighted that in the user's instructions, the manufacturers of Bioplic and Top Comfort did not supply the details of the amount of monomers, initiators, and size of inorganic in their products.

The biocompatibility levels of both of resins were acceptable considering the methodology applied. It is emphasized that this was a laboratory study and an *in vitro* toxic activity cannot imply the same for an *in vivo* application; however, the lack of cytotoxicity can support the clinical safety of a material.

As the cytotoxic effect of the resins was very low after 14 days, we encourage the clinicians not to change the resin covering during every appointment if possible. This will avoid the elution of toxic components from the recently applied covering resin after each orthodontic session.

Table 3 statistical analyses with mean, standard deviation and cell viability values of the experimental groups.

Groups	Mean	SD	Cell viability (%)	Mean	SD	Cell viability (%)	Mean	SD	Cell viability (%)	Mean	SD	Cell viability (%)
	0h			24h			48h			72h		
A	$0.398^{b,c}$	0.033	112.42	0.616^{d}	0.025	87.62	0.571^{d}	0.042	85.22	$0.765^{e,f}$	0.075	93.63
B	0.419^{c}	0.040	118.36	0.065^{a}	0.003	9.24	0.077^{a}	0.004	11.49	0.060^{a}	0.001	7.34
C	$0.393^{b,c}$	0.031	110.01	0.082^{a}	0.007	11.66	0.589^{d}	0.035	87.91	$0.659^{d,e}$	0.122	80.66
D	0.427^{c}	0.053	120.62	0.079^{a}	0.006	11.23	0.561^{d}	0.025	83.73	$0.604^{c,d}$	0.056	73.92
E	0.422^{c}	0.042	119.20	0.071^{a}	0.002	10.09	0.107^{a}	0.017	15.97	0.059^{a}	0.003	7.22
F	0.425^{c}	0.039	120.05	0.356^{c}	0.135	50.64	0.488^{c}	0.068	72.83	$0.519^{b,c}$	0.101	63.52
G	$0.406^{b,c}$	0.040	114.68	0.178^{b}	0.030	25.32	0.355^{b}	0.056	52.98	0.427^{b}	0.132	52.26
H	0.072^{a}	0.010	20.33	$0.132^{a,b}$	0.002	18.77	0.073^{a}	0.008	10.89	0.111^{a}	0.002	13.5
I	0.354^{b}	0.028	100.00	0.703^{e}	0.053	100.00	0.670^{e}	0.090	100.00	0.817^{f}	0.030	100.00
	7days			14days			21days					
A	0.420^{d}	0.022	103.96	0.632^{c}	0.023	81.54	$0.424^{c,d}$	0.046	76.39			
B	0.058^{a}	0.002	14.35	0.116^{a}	0.022	14.96	0.070^{a}	0.007	12.61			
C	0.327^{c}	0.021	80.94	0.626^{c}	0.021	80.77	$0.407^{c,d}$	0.030	73.33			
D	0.335^{c}	0.021	82.92	0.631^{c}	0.011	81.41	$0.410^{c,d}$	0.016	73.87			
E	0.056^{a}	0.002	13.86	0.099^{a}	0.011	12.77	0.092^{a}	0.016	16.57			
F	0.248^{b}	0.102	61.38	$0.645^{c,d}$	0.017	83.22	0.388^{c}	0.022	69.90			
G	$0.382^{c,d}$	0.021	94.55	0.703^{d}	0.041	90.70	0.426^{d}	0.028	76.75			
H	0.087^{a}	0.007	21.53	0.249^{b}	0.030	32.1	0.323^{b}	0.168	58.19			
I	0.404^{d}	0.014	100.00	0.775^{e}	0.111	100.00	0.555^{e}	0.005	100.00			

* SD indicates standard deviation ** Different letters indicate statistical differences at $\alpha = 0.05$

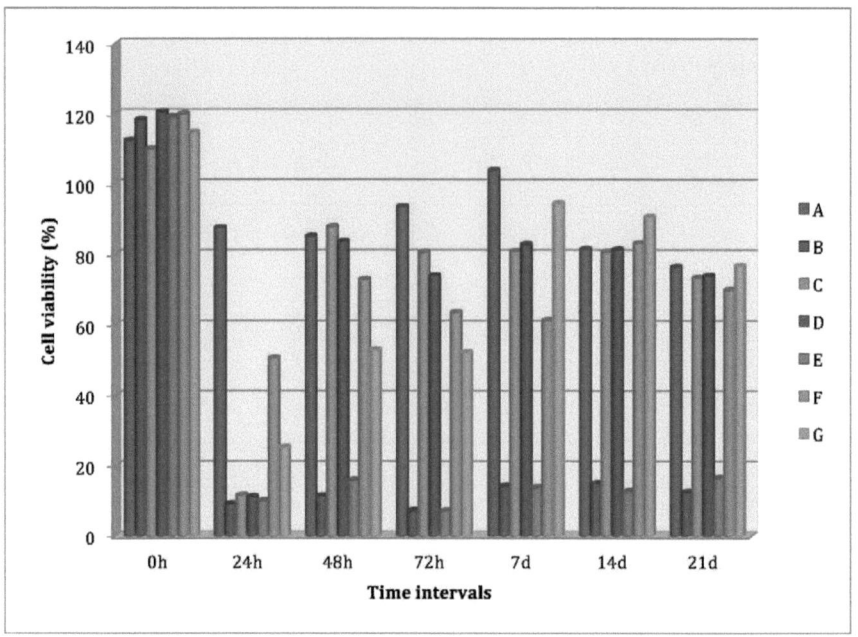

Groups: A - Miniscrew (MS); B - Bioplic as-received; C - Bioplic after light-polymerization; D - Bioplic after light- polymerization placed on MS head; E - Top comfort resin as-received; F - Top comfort after light- polymerization; G - Top comfort after light- polymerization placed on MS head

Figure 17: Percentage of cell viability according to different time intervals until de the end of experiment.

6. *Which resin covering should I use?*

Skeletal anchorage has developed considerably since the first attempts to use rudimentary devices. The flapless surgical technique for placement of miniscrews has brought considerable advancement in patient comfort[41] and acceptance of the temporary anchorage devices. Even with these advances, the use of miniscrews and the orthodontic appliance itself can cause the patient discomfort and pain, and it is the orthodontist's responsibility to try to minimize these side effects.

The aim of this book was to present options of covering resins to improve the patient's comfort and to prevent injuries caused by sharp orthodontic devices. The covering of miniscrew heads was emphasized, but the resins can also be used to cover tubes (Figure 18), jigs (Figure 19), power arms (Figure 20) and other devices that might cause injuries to the soft tissues. We shared our clinical experience and some scientific findings to help the clinician to make his/her choice.

Considering the results of the cytotoxicity assay, although both resins presented acceptable levels of toxicity, Bioplic presented a better performance. On the other hand, the Top Comfort insertion technique is easier (because it has an insertion tip that enables resin deposition directly onto the miniscrew head, and it does not require sculpture), thus demanding little chair time.

We do not intend to persuade the reader to use a specific trademark or product. We encourage orthodontists to test other brands of similar products, such as ProvimasterF (Wilcos, Petrópolis, Rio de Janeiro, Brazil), ClipF (Voco, Cuxhaven, Germany), First Fill (Pentron Clinical Technologies, Wallingford CT, USA) and Soleil (DMG America LLC, Englewood, NJ, USA). We also suggest investigation of the cytotoxic effect of these materials.

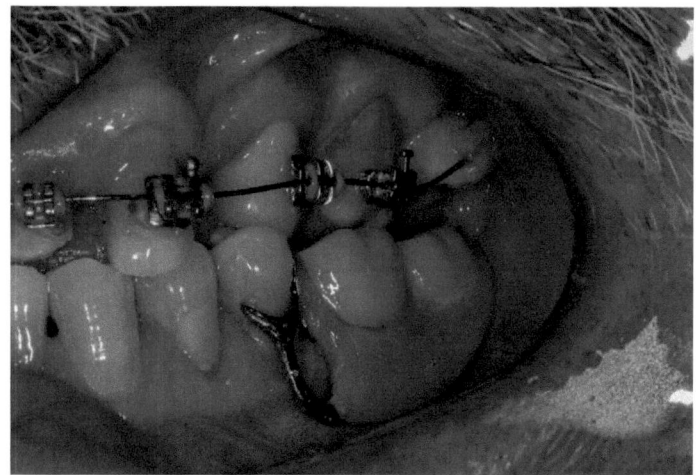

Figure 18: Bioplic was used to cover a tube of a maxillary second molar that was hurting the jugal mucosa at the beginning of its leveling and alignment.

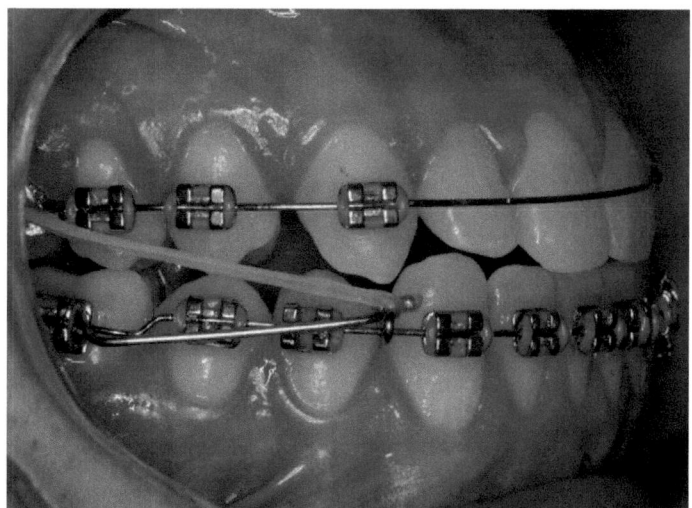

Figure 19: The hook of the sliding jig was covered with Top Comfort.

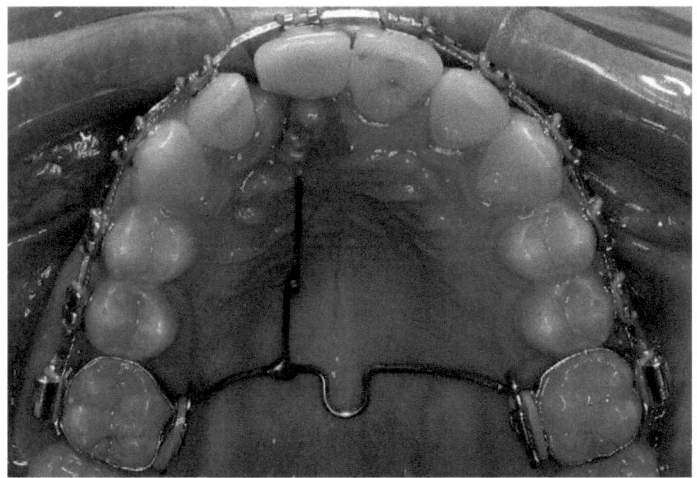

Figure 20: Top comfort covered the ligature and the tip of the power arm used for the traction of the impacted central incisor.

References

1. Angle EH. Treatment of malloclusion of the teeth. Angle's System. 7 ed. Philadelphia: SS White Dental Manufactoring Company; 1907.
2. Melsen B, Verna C. A rational aproach to orthodontic anchorage. Prog Orthod 1999;1:12.
3. Lee JS, Kim JK, Park YC, Vanarsdall Jr RL. Aplicações dos mini-implantes ortodônticos. São Paulo: Quintessence; 2009.
4. Creekmore TD, Eklund MK. The possibility of skeletal anchorage. J Clin Orthod 1983;17(4):266-9.
5. Justens E, De Bruyn H. Clinical outcome of mini-screws used as orthodontic anchorage. Clin Implant Dent Relat Res 2008;10(3):174-80.
6. Block MS, Hoffman DR. A new device for absolute anchorage for orthodontics. Am J Orthod Dentofacial Orthop 1995;107(3):251-8.
7. Wehrbein H, Merz BR, Diedrich P, Glatzmaier J. The use of palatal implants for orthodontic anchorage. Design and clinical application of the orthosystem. Clin Oral Implants Res 1996;7(4):410-6.
8. Melsen B, Petersen JK, Costa A. Zygoma ligatures: an alternative form of maxillary anchorage. J Clin Orthod 1998;32(3):154-8.
9. Umemori M, Sugawara J, Mitani H, Nagasaka H, Kawamura H. Skeletal anchorage system for open-bite correction. Am J Orthod Dentofacial Orthop 1999;115(2):166-74.
10. Kanomi R. Mini-implant for orthodontic anchorage. J Clin Orthod 1997;31(11):763-7.
11. Serra G, Morais LS, Elias CN, et al. Sequential bone healing of immediately loaded mini-implants. Am J Orthod Dentofacial Orthop 2008;134(1):44-52.
12. Luzi C, Verna C, Melsen B. Immediate loading of orthodontic mini-implants: a histomorphometric evaluation of tissue reaction. Eur J Orthod 2009;31(1):21-9.
13. Wei X, Zhao L, Xu Z, Tang T, Zhao Z. Effects of cortical bone thickness at different healing times on microscrew stability. Angle Orthod 2011;81(5):760-6.
14. Topouzelis N, Tsaousoglou P. Clinical factors correlated with the success rate of miniscrews in orthodontic treatment. Int J Oral Sci 2012;4(1):38-44.
15. Papadopoulos MA, Tarawneh F. The use of miniscrew implants for temporary skeletal anchorage in orthodontics: a comprehensive review. Oral Surg Oral Med Oral Pathol Oral Radiol Endod 2007;103(5):e6-15.
16. AlSamak S, Bitsanis E, Makou M, Eliades G. Morphological and structural characteristics of orthodontic mini-implants. J Orofac Orthop 2012;73(1):58-71.

17. Squeff LR, Simonson MBA, Elias CN, Nojima LI. Characterization of mini-implants used for orthodontic anchorage. Dental Press Journal of Orthodontics 2008;13(5):49-56.

18. Javed F, Romanos GE. The role of primary stability for successful immediate loading of dental implants. A literature review. J Dent 2010;38(8):612-20.

19. Gedrange T, Hietschold V, Mai R, et al. An evaluation of resonance frequency analysis for the determination of the primary stability of orthodontic palatal implants. A study in human cadavers. Clin Oral Implants Res 2005;16(4):425-31.

20. Iijima M, Takano M, Yasuda Y, et al. Effect of the quantity and quality of cortical bone on the failure force of a miniscrew implant. Eur J Orthod 2012.

21. Wilmes B, Rademacher C, Olthoff G, Drescher D. Parameters affecting primary stability of orthodontic mini-implants. J Orofac Orthop 2006;67(3):162-74.

22. Cheng SJ, Tseng IY, Lee JJ, Kok SH. A prospective study of the risk factors associated with failure of mini-implants used for orthodontic anchorage. Int J Oral Maxillofac Implants 2004;19(1):100-6.

23. Freudenthaler JW, Haas R, Bantleon HP. Bicortical titanium screws for critical orthodontic anchorage in the mandible: a preliminary report on clinical applications. Clin Oral Implants Res 2001;12(4):358-63.

24. Trisi P, Rao W, Rebaudi A. A histometric comparison of smooth and rough titanium implants in human low-density jawbone. International Journal of Oral Maxillofacial Implants 1999;14(5):689-98.

25. Marquezan M, Mattos CT, Sant'Anna EF, de Souza MM, Maia LC. Does cortical thickness influence the primary stability of miniscrews?: A systematic review and meta-analysis. Angle Orthod 2014;84(6):1093-103.

26. Su YY, Wilmes B, Honscheid R, Drescher D. Application of a wireless resonance frequency transducer to assess primary stability of orthodontic mini-implants: an in vitro study in pig ilia. Int J Oral Maxillofac Implants 2009;24(4):647-54.

27. Marquezan M, Lima I, Lopes RT, Sant'Anna EF, de Souza MM. Is trabecular bone related to primary stability of miniscrews? Angle Orthod 2014;84(3):500-7.

28. Huja SS, Litsky AS, Beck FM, Johnson KA, Larsen PE. Pull-out strength of monocortical screws placed in the maxillae and mandibles of dogs. Am J Orthod Dentofacial Orthop 2005;127(3):307-13.

29. Motoyoshi M, Yoshida T, Ono A, Shimizu N. Effect of cortical bone thickness and implant placement torque on stability of orthodontic mini-implants. Int J Oral Maxillofac Implants 2007;22(5):779-84.

30. Motoyoshi M, Inaba M, Ono A, Ueno S, Shimizu N. The effect of cortical bone thickness on the stability of orthodontic mini-implants and on the stress distribution in surrounding bone. Int J Oral Maxillofac Surg 2009;38(1):13-8.

31. Miyawaki S, Koyama I, Inoue M, et al. Factors associated with the stability of titanium screws placed in the posterior region for orthodontic anchorage. Am J Orthod Dentofacial Orthop 2003;124(4):373-8.

32. Garfinkle JS, Cunningham LL, Jr., Beeman CS, et al. Evaluation of orthodontic mini-implant anchorage in premolar extraction therapy in adolescents. Am J Orthod Dentofacial Orthop 2008;133(5):642-53.

33. Park HS, Jeong SH, Kwon OW. Factors affecting the clinical success of screw implants used as orthodontic anchorage. Am J Orthod Dentofacial Orthop 2006;130(1):18-25.

34. Tweed C. Clinical orthodontics. . Saint Louis: The C.V. Mosby Company.

35. Lee YK, Kim JW, Baek SH, Kim TW, Chang YI. Root and bone response to the proximity of a mini-implant under orthodontic loading. Angle Orthod 2010;80(3):452-8.

36. Kravitz ND, Kusnoto B. Risks and complications of orthodontic miniscrews. Am J Orthod Dentofacial Orthop 2007;131(4 Suppl):S43-51.

37. Fabbroni G, Aabed S, Mizen K, Starr DG. Transalveolar screws and the incidence of dental damage: a prospective study. Int J Oral Maxillofac Surg 2004;33(5):442-6.

38. Kim JW, Ahn SJ, Chang YI. Histomorphometric and mechanical analyses of the drill-free screw as orthodontic anchorage. Am J Orthod Dentofacial Orthop 2005;128(2):190-4.

39. Kadioglu O, Buyukyilmaz T, Zachrisson BU, Maino BG. Contact damage to root surfaces of premolars touching miniscrews during orthodontic treatment. Am J Orthod Dentofacial Orthop 2008;134(3):353-60.

40. Kuroda S, Yamada K, Deguchi T, et al. Root proximity is a major factor for screw failure in orthodontic anchorage. Am J Orthod Dentofacial Orthop 2007;131(4 Suppl):S68-73.

41. Kuroda S, Tanaka E. Risks and complications of miniscrew anchorage in clinical orthodontics. Japanese Dental Science Review 2014;50:79-85.

42. da Cunha AC, Marquezan M, Lima I, et al. Influence of bone architecture on the primary stability of different mini-implant designs. Am J Orthod Dentofacial Orthop 2015;147(1):45-51.

43. Melsen B. Mini-implants: Where are we? J Clin Orthod 2005;39(9):539-47; quiz 31-2.

44. Heidemann W, Terheyden H, Louis Gerlach K. Analysis of the osseous/metal interface of drill free screws and self-tapping screws. J Maxillofac Surg 2001;29(2):69-74.

45. Kesling P. Questions and miniscrews. J Clin Orthod 2005;39(9):527-8; author reply 28-30.

46. Teughels W, Van Assche N, Sliepen I, Quirynen M. Effect of material characteristics and/or surface topography on biofilm development. Clin Oral Implants Res 2006;17 Suppl 2:68-81.

47. Quirynen M, Bollen CM, Papaioannou W, Van Eldere J, van Steenberghe D. The influence of titanium abutment surface roughness on plaque accumulation and gingivitis: short-term observations. Int J Oral Maxillofac Implants 1996;11(2):169-78.

48. Osório AAF. Microbiological aspects associated with orthodontic mini-implants [Rio de Janeiro: Federal University of Rio de Janeiro; 2014.

49. Marquezan M, de Freitas AO, Nojima LI. Miniscrew covering: an alternative to prevent traumatic lesions. Am J Orthod Dentofacial Orthop 2012;141(2):242-4.

50. Graber LW, Vanarsdall Jr. RL, Vig KWL. Orthodontics: Current Principles and Techniques. 5th Edition ed: Elsevier; 2012.

51. Proffit WR, Fields HF, Sarver DM. Contemporary Orthodontics. 5th Edition ed: Elsevier; 2012.

52. Gainsforth BL, LB H. A study of orthodontic anchorage possibilities in basal bone. American Journal of Orthodontics and Oral Surgery. 1945;31(8):11.

53. Sherman AJ. Bone reaction to orthodontic forces on vitreous carbon dental implants. Am J Orthod 1978;74(1):79-87.

54. Turley PK, Shapiro PA, Moffett BC. The loading of bioglass-coated aluminium oxide implants to produce sutural expansion of the maxillary complex in the pigtail monkey (Macaca nemestrina). Arch Oral Biol 1980;25(7):459-69.

55. Ismail SF, Johal AS. The role of implants in orthodontics. J Orthod 2002;29(3):239-45.

56. Roberts WE, Helm FR, Marshall KJ, Gongloff RK. Rigid endosseous implants for orthodontic and orthopedic anchorage. Angle Orthod 1989;59(4):247-56.

57. Roberts WE, Marshall KJ, Mozsary PG. Rigid endosseous implant utilized as anchorage to protract molars and close an atrophic extraction site. Angle Orthod 1990;60(2):135-52.

58. Brånemark PI. Osseointegration and its experimental background. . Journal of Prosthetic Dentistry 1983;50(3):399-410.

59. Albrektsson T, Johansson C. Osteoinduction, osteoconduction and osseointegration. Eur Spine J 2001;10 Suppl 2:S96-101.

60. Huang LH, Shotwell JL, Wang HL. Dental implants for orthodontic anchorage. Am J Orthod Dentofacial Orthop 2005;127(6):713-22.

61. Wahl N. Orthodontics in 3 millennia. Chapter 15: Skeletal anchorage. Am J Orthod Dentofacial Orthop 2008;134(5):707-10.

62. Alves JR M, Baratieri C, Marquezan M, et al. Palate: What to know before mini-implant's placement? Rev Clín Ortod Dental Press 2012;11(1):108-14.

63. De Clerck H, Geerinckx V, Siciliano S. The Zygoma Anchorage System. J Clin Orthod 2002;36(8):455-9.

64. Sugawara J. Temporary skeletal anchorage devices: the case for miniplates. Am J Orthod Dentofacial Orthop 2014;145(5):559-65.

65. Mah J, Bergstrand F. Temporary anchorage devices: a status report. J Clin Orthod 2005;39(3):132-6; discussion 36; quiz 53.

66. Eroglu T, Kaya B, Cetinsahin A, Arman A, Uckan S. Success of zygomatic plate-screw anchorage system. J Oral Maxillofac Surg 2010;68(3):602-5.

67. De Clerck EE, Swennen GR. Success rate of miniplate anchorage for bone anchored maxillary protraction. Angle Orthod 2011;81(6):1010-3.

68. Schatzle M, Mannchen R, Zwahlen M, Lang NP. Survival and failure rates of orthodontic temporary anchorage devices: a systematic review. Clin Oral Implants Res 2009;20(12):1351-9.

69. Baumgaertel S. Temporary skeletal anchorage devices: the case for miniscrews. Am J Orthod Dentofacial Orthop 2014;145(5):558-64.

70. Tseng YC, Chen CM, Wang HC, et al. Pain perception during miniplate-assisted orthodontic therapy. Kaohsiung J Med Sci 2010;26(11):603-8.

71. Lim JE, Lee SJ, Kim YJ, Lim WH, Chun YS. Comparison of cortical bone thickness and root proximity at maxillary and mandibular interradicular sites for orthodontic mini-implant placement. Orthod Craniofac Res 2009;12(4):299-304.

72. Schnelle MA, Beck FM, Jaynes RM, Huja SS. A radiographic evaluation of the availability of bone for placement of miniscrews. Angle Orthod 2004;74(6):832-7.

73. Stanford N. Mini-screws success rates sufficient for orthodontic treatment. Evid Based Dent 2011;12(1):19.

74. Reynders R, Ronchi L, Bipat S. Mini-implants in orthodontics: a systematic review of the literature. Am J Orthod Dentofacial Orthop 2009;135(5):564 e1-19; discussion 64-5.

75. Kuroda S, Sugawara Y, Deguchi T, Kyung HM, Takano-Yamamoto T. Clinical use of miniscrew implants as orthodontic anchorage: success rates and postoperative discomfort. Am J Orthod Dentofacial Orthop 2007;131(1):9-15.

76. Wiechmann D, Meyer U, Buchter A. Success rate of mini- and micro-implants used for orthodontic anchorage: a prospective clinical study. Clin Oral Implants Res 2007;18(2):263-7.

77. Park HS, Lee YJ, Jeong SH, Kwon TG. Density of the alveolar and basal bones of the maxilla and the mandible. Am J Orthod Dentofacial Orthop 2008;133(1):30-7.

78. Motoyoshi M, Matsuoka M, Shimizu N. Application of orthodontic mini-implants in adolescents. Int J Oral Maxillofac Surg 2007;36(8):695-9.

79. Okazaki J, Komasa Y, Sakai D, et al. A torque removal study on the primary stability of orthodontic titanium screw mini-implants in the cortical bone of dog femurs. Int J Oral Maxillofac Surg 2008;37(7):647-50.

80. Buchter A, Wiechmann D, Koerdt S, et al. Load-related implant reaction of mini-implants used for orthodontic anchorage. Clin Oral Implants Res 2005;16(4):473-9.

81. Lim SA, Cha JY, Hwang CJ. Insertion torque of orthodontic miniscrews according to changes in shape, diameter and length. Angle Orthod 2008;78(2):234-40.

82. Marquezan M, Lau TC, Mattos CT, et al. Bone mineral density. Angle Orthod 2012;82(1):62-6.

83. Wilmes B, Drescher D. Impact of insertion depth and predrilling diameter on primary stability of orthodontic mini-implants. Angle Orthod 2009;79(4):609-14.

84. Brinley CL, Behrents R, Kim KB, et al. Pitch and longitudinal fluting effects on the primary stability of miniscrew implants. Angle Orthod 2009;79(6):1156-61.

85. Cunha AC, Marquezan M, Lima I, et al. Influence of bone architecture on the primary stability of different mini-implant designs. Am J Orthod Dentofacial Orthop 2015;147(1):45-51.

86. Walter A, Winsauer H, Marcé-Nogué J, Mojal S, Puigdollers A. Design characteristics, primary stability and risk of fracture of orthodontic mini-implants: pilot scan electron microscope and mechanical studies. Med Oral Patol Oral Cir Bucal 2013;18(5):e804-10.

87. Monga N, Chaurasia S, Kharbanda OP, Duggal R, Rajeswari MR. A study of interleukin 1beta levels in peri-miniscrew crevicular fluid (PMCF). Prog Orthod 2014;15(1):30.

88.	Enhos S, Veli I, Cakmak O, et al. OPG and RANKL levels around miniscrew implants during orthodontic tooth movement. Am J Orthod Dentofacial Orthop 2013;144(2):203-9.

89.	Nienkemper M, Wilmes B, Pauls A, Drescher D. Impact of mini-implant length on stability at the initial healing period: a controlled clinical study. Head Face Med 2013;9:30.

90.	Nienkemper M, Wilmes B, Pauls A, Drescher D. Mini-implant stability at the initial healing period: a clinical pilot study. Angle Orthod 2014;84(1):127-33.

91.	Lehnen S, McDonald F, Bourauel C, Baxmann M. Patient expectations, acceptance and preferences in treatment with orthodontic mini-implants. A randomly controlled study. Part I: insertion techniques. J Orofac Orthop 2011;72(2):93-102.

92.	Baxmann M, McDonald F, Bourauel C, Jager A. Expectations, acceptance, and preferences regarding microimplant treatment in orthodontic patients: A randomized controlled trial. Am J Orthod Dentofacial Orthop 2010;138(3):250 e1-50 e10; discussion 50-1.

93.	Kvam E, Bondevik O, Gjerdet NR. Traumatic ulcers and pain in adults during orthodontic treatment. Community Dent Oral Epidemiol 1989;17(3):154-7.

94.	Oh JS, Kim SG. Clinical study of the relationship between implant stability measurements using Periotest and Osstell mentor and bone quality assessment. Oral Surg Oral Med Oral Pathol Oral Radiol 2012;113(3):e35-40.

95.	Chaddad K, Ferreira AF, Geurs N, Reddy MS. Influence of surface characteristics on survival rates of mini-implants. Angle Orthod 2008;78(1):107-13.

96.	Caulier H, Naert I, Kalk W, Jansen JA. The relationship of some histologic parameters, radiographic evaluations, and Periotest measurements of oral implants: an experimental animal study. Int J Oral Maxillofac Implants 1997;12(3):380-6.

97.	Lehnen S, McDonald F, Bourauel C, Jager A, Baxmann M. Expectations, acceptance and preferences of patients in treatment with orthodontic mini-implants: part II: implant removal. J Orofac Orthop 2011;72(3):214-22.

98.	Cehreli S, Yilmaz A, Arman-Ozcirpici A. Cortical bone strains around straight and angulated immediate orthodontic microimplants: a pilot study. Implant Dent 2013;22(2):133-7.

99.	Zawawi KH. Acceptance of orthodontic miniscrews as temporary anchorage devices. Patient Prefer Adherence 2014;8:933-7.

100.	Subramani K, Jung RE, Molenberg A, Hammerle CH. Biofilm on dental implants: a review of the literature. Int J Oral Maxillofac Implants 2009;24(4):616-26.

101. Al-Ahmad A, Wiedmann-Al-Ahmad M, Fackler A, et al. In vivo study of the initial bacterial adhesion on different implant materials. Arch Oral Biol 2013;58(9):1139-47.
102. Shehata M, Durner J, Eldenez A, et al. Cytotoxicity and induction of DNA double-strand breaks by components leached from dental composites in primary human gingival fibroblasts. Dent Mater 2013;29(9):971-9.
103. Ausiello P, Cassese A, Miele C, et al. Cytotoxicity of dental resin composites: an in vitro evaluation. J Appl Toxicol 2013;33(6):451-7.
104. Jorge JH, Giampaolo ET, Machado AL, Vergani CE. Cytotoxicity of denture base acrylic resins: a literature review. J Prosthet Dent 2003;90(2):190-3.
105. Hensten-Pettersen A. Skin and mucosal reactions associated with dental materials. Eur J Oral Sci 1998;106(2 Pt 2):707-12.
106. Goncalves TS, Morganti MA, Campos LC, Rizzatto SM, Menezes LM. Allergy to auto-polymerized acrylic resin in an orthodontic patient. Am J Orthod Dentofacial Orthop 2006;129(3):431-5.
107. Goncalves TS, de Menezes LM, Silva LE. Residual monomer of autopolymerized acrylic resin according to different manipulation and polishing methods. An in situ evaluation. Angle Orthod 2008;78(4):722-7.
108. Malkoc S, Corekci B, Ulker HE, Yalcin M, Sengun A. Cytotoxic effects of orthodontic composites. Angle Orthod 2010;80(4):571-6.
109. Malkoc S, Corekci B, Botsali HE, Yalcin M, Sengun A. Cytotoxic effects of resin-modified orthodontic band adhesives. Are they safe? Angle Orthod 2010;80(5):890-5.
110. Pithon MM, dos Santos RL, Martins FO, Romanos MTV, Araújo MTS. Evaluation of Cytotoxicity and Degree of Conversion of Orthodontic Adhesives over Different Time Periods. Materials Research. 2010;13(2):165-69.
111. dos Santos GL, Beltrame AP, Triches TC, et al. Analysis of microleakage of temporary restorative materials in primary teeth. J Indian Soc Pedod Prev Dent 2014;32(2):130-4.
112. Borefreund E, Puerner A. A simple quantitative procedure using monolayer cultures for cytotoxic assays (HTD/NR90). Journal of Tissue Culture Methods. 1984;9(1):7-9.
113. Geurtsen W, Lehmann F, Spahl W, Leyhausen G. Cytotoxicity of 35 dental resin composite monomers/additives in permanent 3T3 and three human primary fibroblast cultures. J Biomed Mater Res 1998;41(3):474-80.
114. Stanislawski L, Lefeuvre M, Bourd K, et al. TEGDMA-induced toxicity in human fibroblasts is associated with early and drastic glutathione depletion

with subsequent production of oxygen reactive species. J Biomed Mater Res A 2003;66(3):476-82.

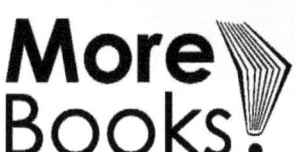
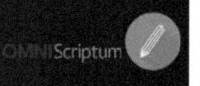

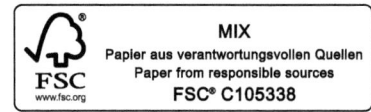

Printed by Books on Demand GmbH, Norderstedt / Germany